Helen Keller

OTHER BIOGRAPHIES AVAILABLE IN YEARLING BOOKS:

Maria Tallchief, ADELE DE LEEUW

Harriet Tubman, SAM AND BERYL EPSTEIN

Cesar Chavez, FLORENCE M. WHITE

William C. Handy, ELIZABETH RIDER MONTGOMERY

Martin Luther King, Jr., LILLIE PATTERSON

Sitting Bull, LAVERE ANDERSON

Chief Joseph, ELIZABETH RIDER MONTGOMERY

Robert F. Kennedy, CHARLES P. GRAVES

Frederick Douglass, LILLIE PATTERSON

Helen Keller, STEWART AND POLLY ANN GRAFF

Helen Keller
Toward the Light

by Stewart and Polly Anne Graff

illustrated by Paul Frame

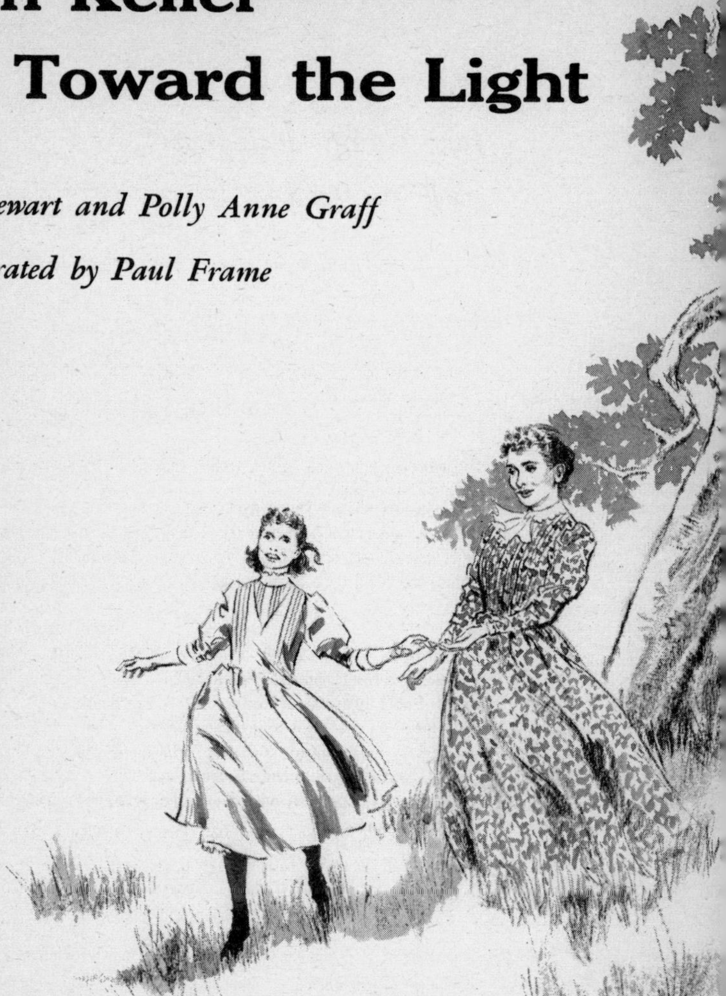

A YEARLING BOOK

This book is for
Jane Campbell Harris
with our love

Published by
DELL PUBLISHING CO., INC.
1 Dag Hammarskjold Plaza
New York, N.Y. 10017

ISBN: 0-440-43566-8

Reprinted by arrangement with Garrard Publishing Company.
Printed in U. S. A.
Seventeenth Dell Printing—May 1977
HELEN KELLER is one of the *Discovery* biographies published by Garrard Publishing Co., Champaign, Illinois.
Discovery books are published by Garrard in library bindings.

This book is one of a series of educational, informative biographies, presented in a lively, colorful and interesting manner. They are designed and edited so that they can be read and enjoyed by young readers through the elementary grades. All facts are authentic for they have been carefully checked with leading sources for historical accuracy.

Contents

Helen Keller: Toward the Light

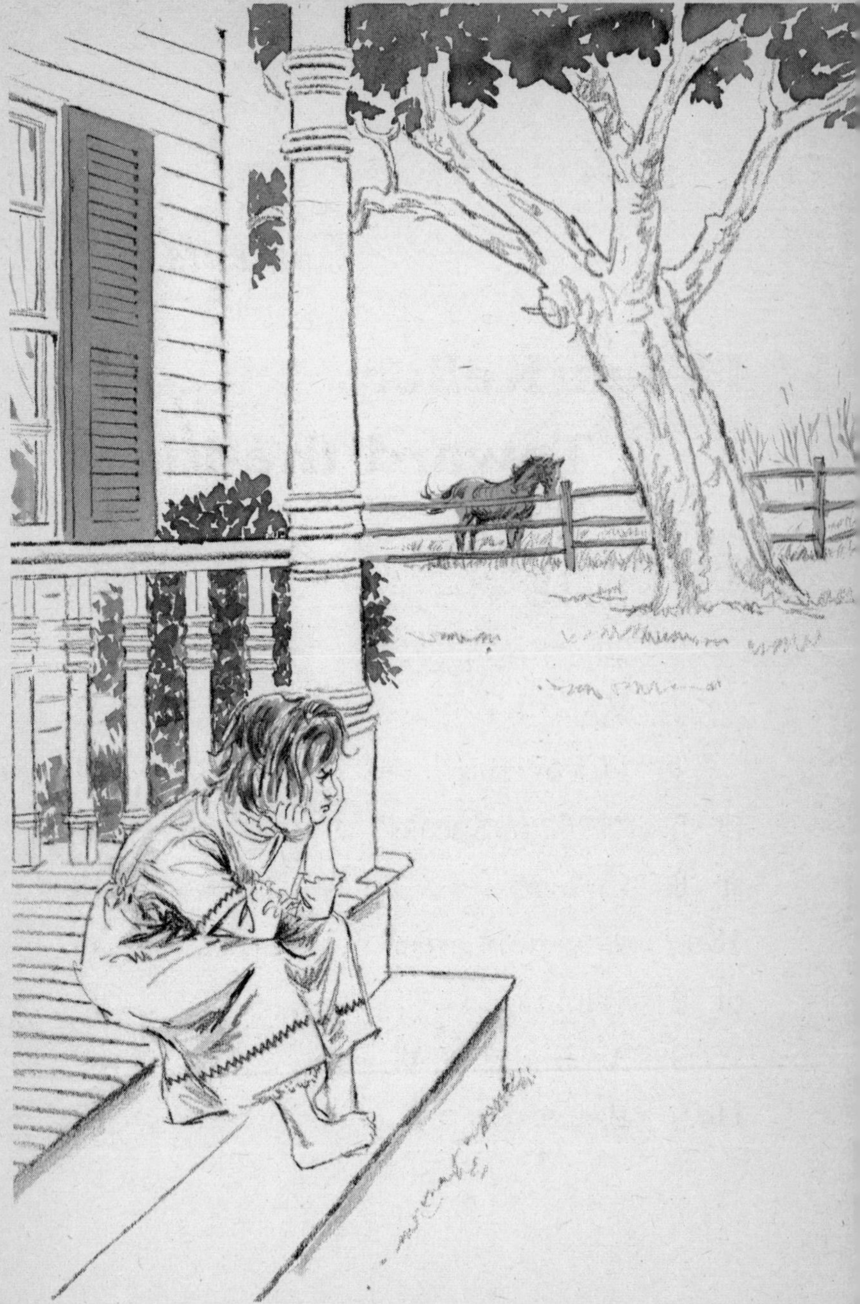

Chapter 1

Darkness

One afternoon a little girl sat on the porch steps of her home. It was her sixth birthday, June 27, in the year 1886. The house was in the small town of Tuscumbia, Alabama.

The little girl had curly golden hair. Her bare arms and legs were sturdy.

But there was something strange about her eyes. When she stared into the bright sun she did not blink.

Roses bloomed in the arbor. Across the yard, a pony whinnied in the pasture. It would have been a nice afternoon to ride, but the little girl sat alone. There was a queer, angry expression on her face.

She could feel the warm sun, but she could not see anything but blackness, because she was blind. She could smell the roses, but she could not see their color. She could not hear her pony whinny, because she was deaf also.

The little girl's name was Helen Keller. She lived with her parents and her baby sister Mildred in a comfortable house with wide fields and a big barn.

Helen's father had been a captain in the Civil War. Now he owned a newspaper.

When Helen Keller was born she could see and hear like other children. But when she was a year and a half old she became very ill. Fever burned her small body. The doctors could not help. Her mother and father were afraid Helen would die.

At last Helen got better, but the fever left a terrible mark. When her mother brought a lamp, Helen did not look at the bright light. When her father clapped his hands loudly, she did not turn toward the sound. Then they knew that their little girl was blind and deaf.

Helen was soon well and strong again. When she grew older she wanted to run and play. But when she ran she crashed into trees and fences or fell and hurt herself.

Other children were afraid to play with her because she often hit them roughly and broke their toys. Even Belle, the family's setter dog, ran away from her. Helen did not understand that anyone had feelings except herself. Once she pushed her baby sister out of her cradle.

Worst of all, Helen could not speak or understand others. Her mind was bright and active. She could feel her way quickly through the house or follow the path to the barn. She learned a few signs. She would pull or push to mean "come" or "go." She could show her mother that she was hungry or thirsty.

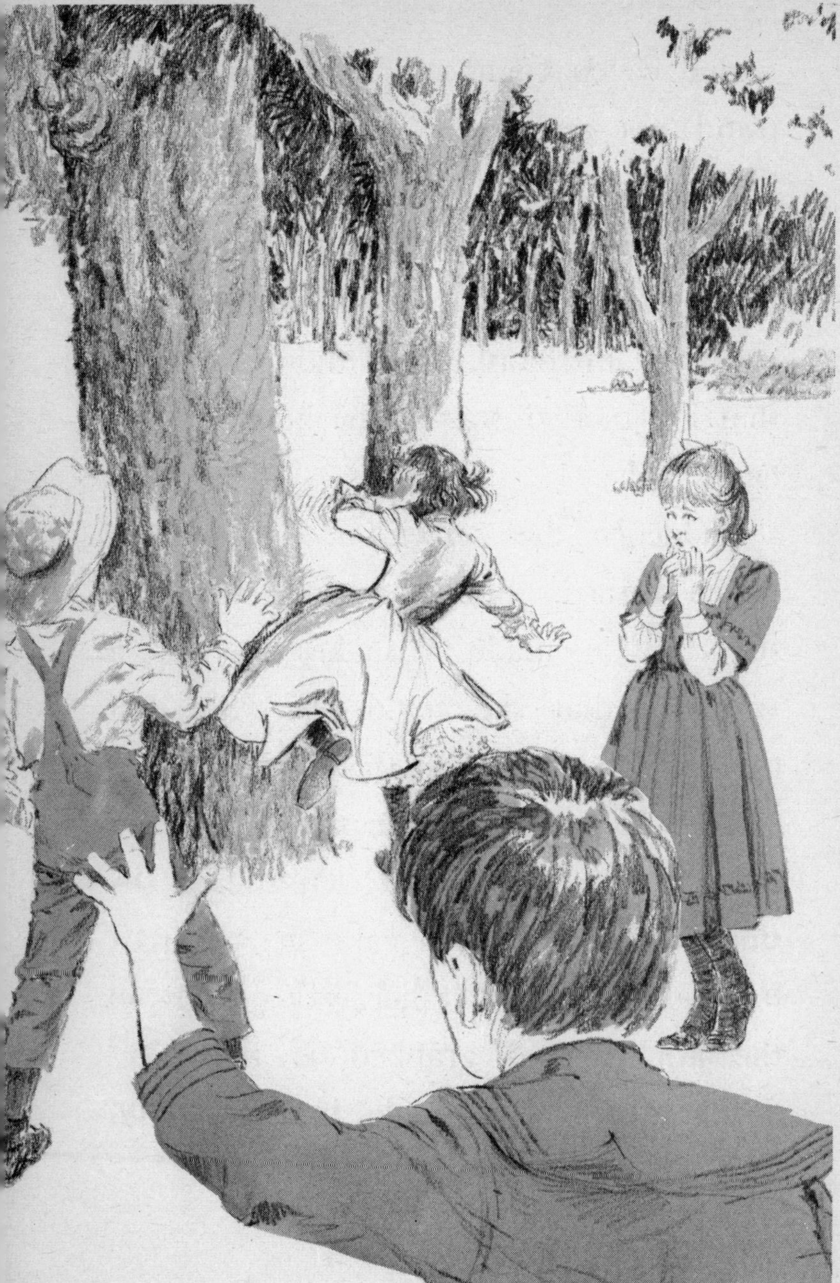

But Helen could not hear voices. She could not see people talking. She did not know that people talked in *words.*

Sitting on the porch steps, Helen was restless and lonely. She did not know it was her birthday. She did not know that her mother was in the house baking her a cake.

Suddenly the screen door slammed. Helen turned. She could not *hear* the slam but it made a shake. It was a *vibration* that she could *feel.* She felt the tap-tap of her mother's footsteps.

Mrs. Keller had come to dress Helen for supper. But when Helen sniffed the smell of freshly baked cake she ran past her mother. She felt her way quickly to the kitchen and grabbed at the cake. She stuffed warm chunks in her mouth.

Mrs. Keller hurried after Helen. She took the cake away, and put it out of reach.

Helen was angry. She loved sweets and she was used to eating anything she wanted. She did not know the cake was for her birthday supper. She kicked and screamed. She fell on the floor sobbing.

Before her mother could stop her Helen rushed outdoors. She ran wildly into a bramble bush. The thorns scraped her face. She tripped and fell. A sharp stone cut her knee.

Mrs. Keller carried Helen back inside. She bandaged Helen's knee and put her to bed. The birthday cake was spoiled. Helen was worn out with temper and crying. She was alone in the darkness again.

Downstairs Helen's mother and father ate their supper sadly. Mrs. Keller told her husband what had just happened. "Helen's tempers are growing worse," Mrs. Keller said.

"But we cannot punish her when she does not understand." Captain Keller shook his head. "If only we could find someone who could help her."

Chapter 2

The Stranger

One morning soon afterward Helen woke early. She could not see the daylight, but she smelled bacon cooking. She knew it was time to get up. Her mother hurried Helen through breakfast and dressed her carefully.

Helen did not know what was happening. Still she felt excited. When her father lifted her into the carriage she wondered where they were going.

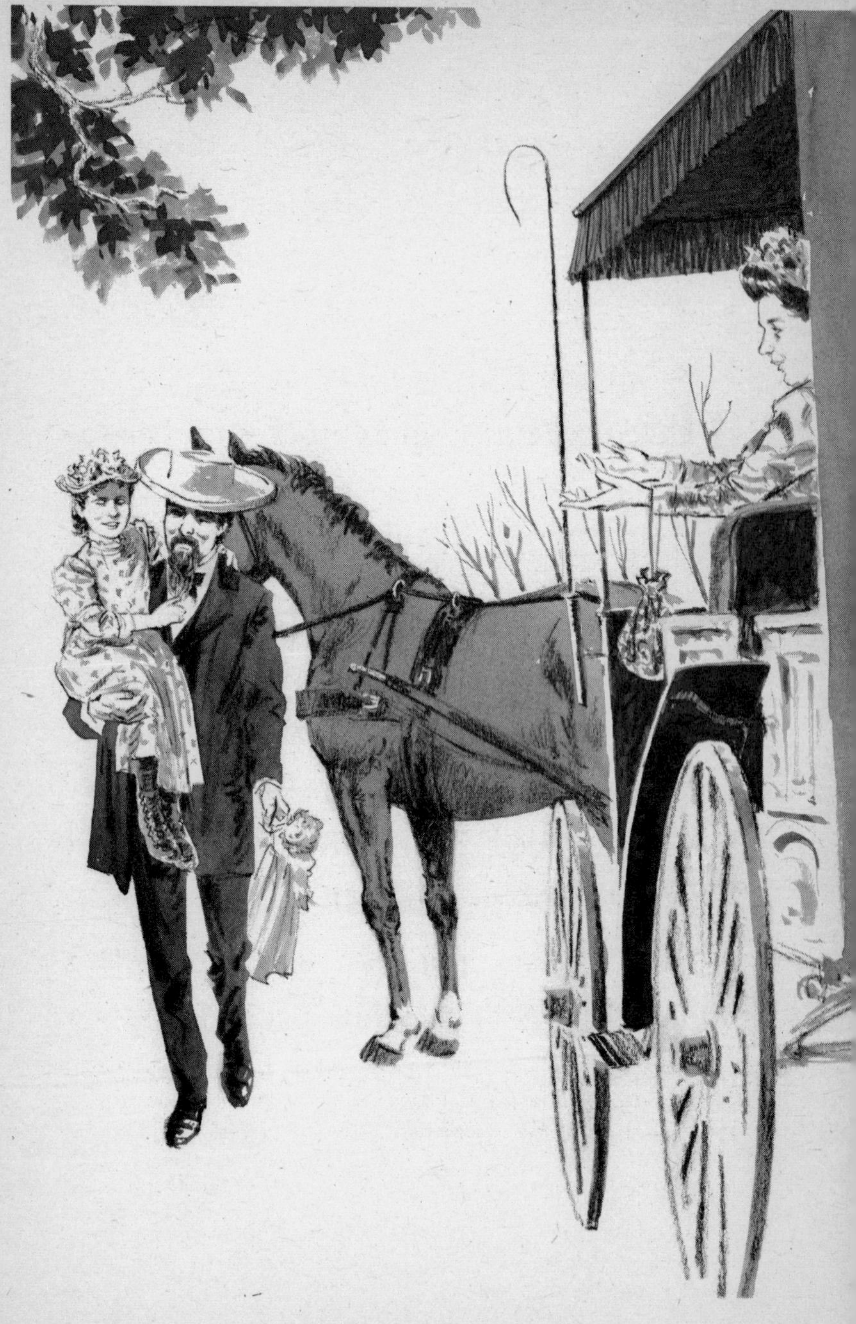

Soon they were on a train. Helen did not understand the strange rumble of the wheels. But she could *feel* that they were moving. She could feel the train rocking and swaying. When the whistle blew she could feel the vibration.

Helen's mother and father were taking her on a long trip to Baltimore, in Maryland. They took her to a famous doctor who had helped many blind children. They hoped he could help Helen.

After the doctor had tested Helen's eyes and ears he shook his head. "Helen will always be blind and deaf," he told her parents. "But she is very intelligent. She can learn. Perhaps Dr. Alexander Graham Bell can help you find someone to teach her."

The Kellers went to Washington to see Dr. Bell. He was famous as the inventor of the telephone. He had spent many years working to help deaf people.

Helen did not know why they made another visit. She did not know the kind man who held her on his knee. She touched his face and felt his gentle smile. He let Helen hold his watch against her cheek. She could feel it tick.

Dr. Bell told Captain Keller about a school for blind children in Boston, Massachusetts. It was called the Perkins Institute.

"There was a girl named Laura Bridgeman who was blind and deaf," Dr. Bell said. "Dr. Howe at the Perkins school taught her to understand words by spelling with his fingers. He pressed the letters against her hand and showed her how to make each letter of the alphabet with her own fingers. Dr. Howe is dead. You must write to Dr. Anagnos at the Perkins school. Ask him to find a teacher who will help Helen."

After the journey home to Alabama, Helen lived in the same dark world again. Her mind was like a wild bird in a cage. She still flew into terrible tempers. She did not know that her mother and father were hoping that Dr. Anagnos could send a teacher for her.

Many months passed. Then one spring day Helen felt excitement in the house again. All day she grew more curious. She waited on the front porch until at last she felt the thud of the horse's hoofs in the drive. The carriage stopped.

There was a thump as a heavy suitcase was set down.

Helen felt new footsteps coming toward her. Her curiosity was bursting. She rushed at the stranger and felt a young woman's arms go around her. Helen's fingers flew over the new face and clothes and handbag.

The stranger had a nice, smiling face. She took Helen's hand and led her upstairs. Soon Helen was helping the stranger unpack. She found a doll. From the stranger's signs she understood that it was a present for her.

Helen hugged the doll. Then she felt the stranger take her hand and make queer signs in it with her fingers. Helen felt the same signs over and over. The stranger was making the letters that

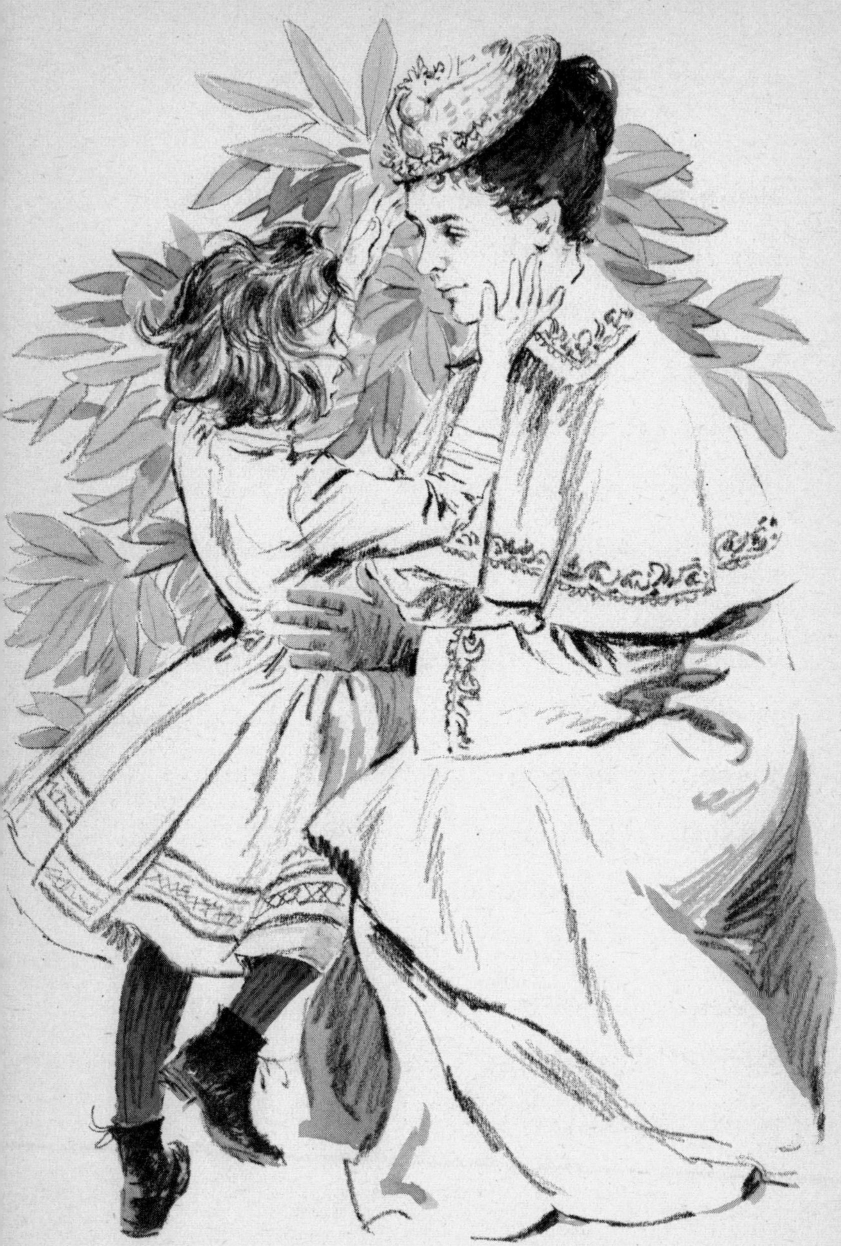

spelled "D-O-L-L." She was showing Helen her very first word in the finger alphabet, but Helen did not understand. Helen was frightened. She threw the doll away and ran to find her mother.

The stranger was a young woman named Anne Sullivan. Dr. Anagnos had sent Anne from the Perkins school in Boston. Anne had been a pupil in the school. She had been almost blind herself. But her blindness was not the same as Helen's. When she was sixteen, an operation helped her to see again.

Now Anne was 21. Her eyes were still weak, but she had started out to earn her living. She had come to Tuscumbia to be Helen Keller's teacher. Soon "Miss Annie" was a new member of the family.

Chapter 3

W-a-t-e-r

The next weeks were an adventure for Helen. She liked the sewing cards and the kindergarten beads that Annie gave her. She liked their long walks through the cool woods. They rode horseback together. Annie led Helen's pony.

Whatever they did Annie spelled letters into Helen's hand. When they petted the cat Annie spelled "C-A-T."

Helen quickly learned to imitate Annie's fingers. She could make the letters for "C-A-K-E" when she wanted a treat, and "M-I-L-K" when she was thirsty.

"Helen is like a clever little monkey," Annie wrote. "She has learned the *signs* to ask for what she wants but she has no idea that she is spelling *words*."

Helen enjoyed the adventures with Annie. But she did not know that the stranger was her teacher. She was very unhappy when Annie tried to make her obey.

Annie did not believe that Helen's parents were right to let Helen always do exactly as she pleased. At mealtimes Helen walked around the table. She dipped her fingers into everyone's plates and gobbled whatever she wanted.

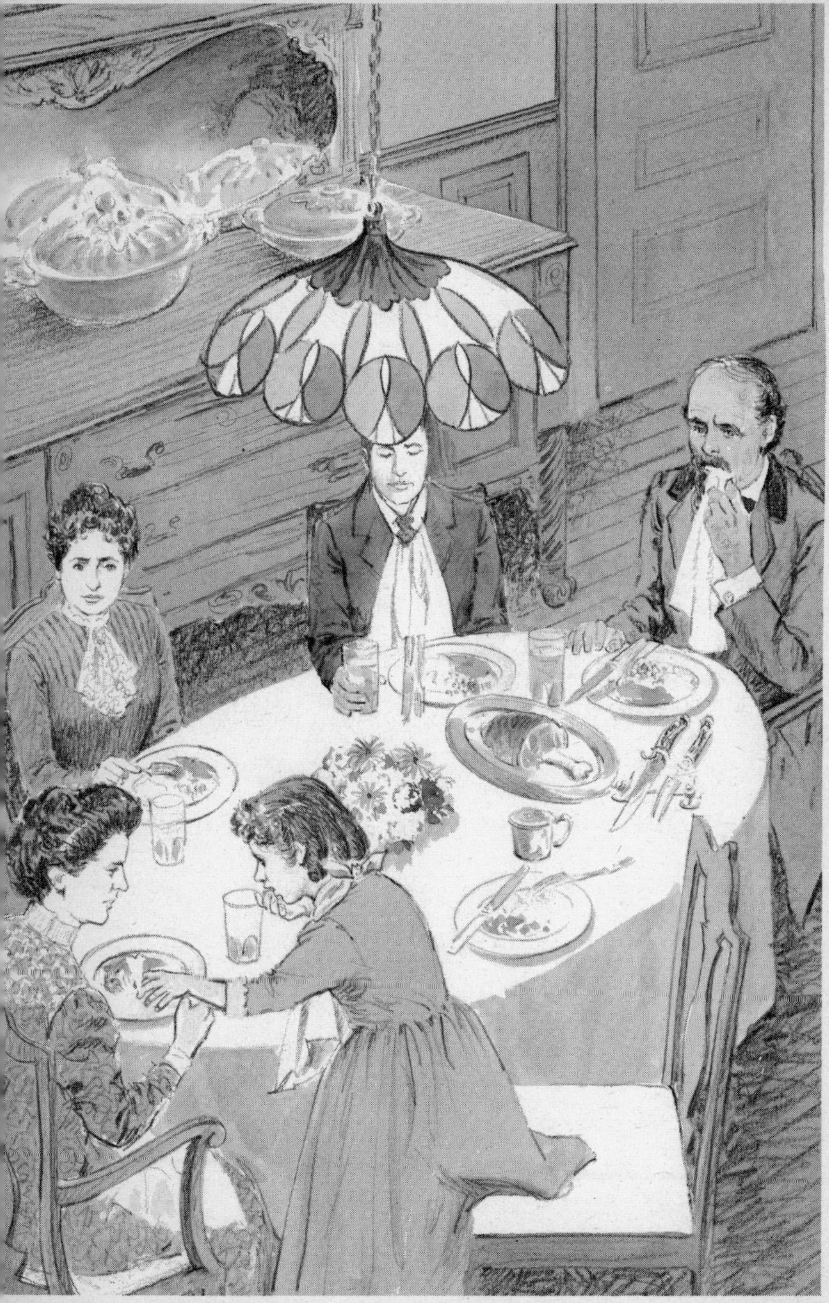

Annie made Helen sit in her own chair and eat from her own plate. Helen was furious. When Annie gave her a spoon, Helen threw it on the floor and kicked the table. They spent a whole afternoon fighting while Annie insisted that Helen fold her napkin.

Mrs. Keller was upset. "I cannot bear to have Helen punished," she said.

Annie was firm. "We must make Helen know we love her," she said. "But we must not let her think she is different because she is blind and deaf. She must behave like other children."

Helen's bad tempers went on. Once she locked Annie in her room and hid the key. Captain Keller had to put a ladder up to Annie's window and help her down.

One morning during her lesson Helen was especially bad. She slammed her new doll on the floor and broke it. Annie was too tired to go on with the lesson. Her eyes ached. She took Helen by the hand and led her outdoors. They stopped at the pump for a drink.

Then something happened that changed Helen's whole life.

Helen held her hand under the spout while Annie pumped. As cold water poured over Helen's hand, Annie spelled in her other hand "W-A-T-E-R." A new expression came into Helen's face. She spelled *water* several times herself. Then she pointed to the ground. Annie quickly spelled "G-R-O-U-N-D."

Helen jumped up. She suddenly realized that she was understanding

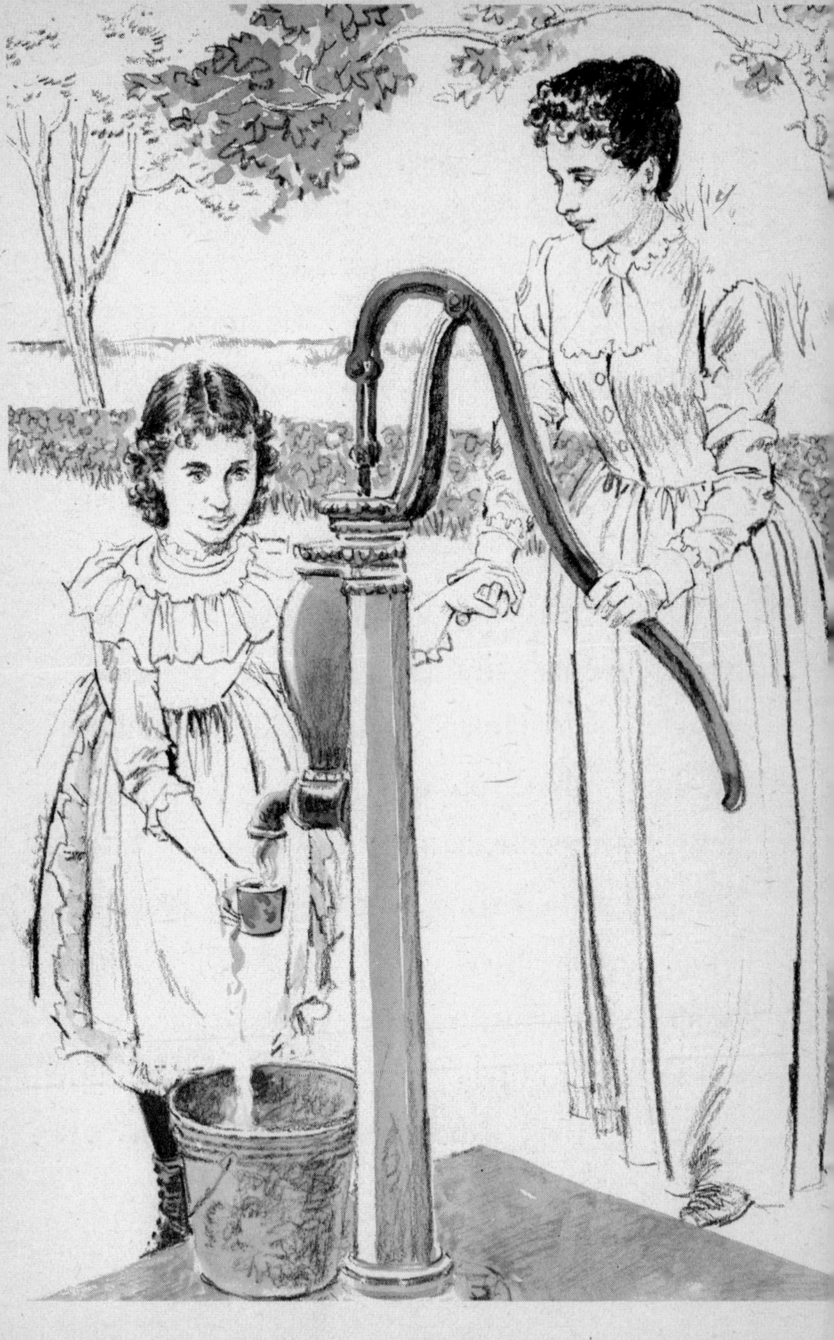

words. She pointed to Annie, and Annie spelled "T-E-A-C-H-E-R." Helen never called Annie by any other name.

Then Helen pointed to herself and Annie slowly spelled out "H-E-L-E-N K-E-L-L-E-R."

Helen's face broke into a wide smile. It was the first time she knew that she had a name.

Helen and Annie were both excited. They raced to the house to find Mrs. Keller. Helen threw herself in her mother's arms while Annie spelled "M-O-T-H-E-R" into her hand. When Helen nodded to show that she understood there were tears of happiness in Mrs. Keller's eyes.

All the rest of the day Helen ran about touching things and Annie spelled the names. When she touched her little sister, Annie spelled "B-A-B-Y."

At supper Annie rubbed her fingers. "No wonder my hand is numb from spelling," she said, smiling at Captain Keller. "Helen is trying to make up in one day what other children have taken six years to learn."

When Helen went to bed that night she kissed her teacher for the first time. Annie wrote, "I thought my heart would burst with joy."

Helen herself said many years later, "I was born again that day. I had been a little ghost in a *no-world*. Now I knew my name. I was a person. I could understand people and make them understand me."

Chapter **4**

Discoveries

Soon Helen could spell enough words to ask questions. She wanted to know what her mother and father and sister and teacher looked like. She learned that Annie had black hair and pretty blue eyes. Annie had a merry Irish wit and she taught Helen to love laughter.

Helen's days were happy that summer. Every morning she and Annie had lessons. Annie made maps out of clay. Helen could feel the shapes of mountains and rivers and continents. Annie gave Helen an orange to hold when she explained that the world was round. When the lesson was over Helen held up the orange and laughed. "Now we can eat the world," she spelled.

Helen learned to count with wooden beads and straws. She touched trees and flowers and learned their names. She held an egg in her hand and felt a baby chick peck its way out. She put her hand in a bowl of water and felt tadpoles swim between her fingers.

One morning there was a surprise for Helen. Annie gave her several square

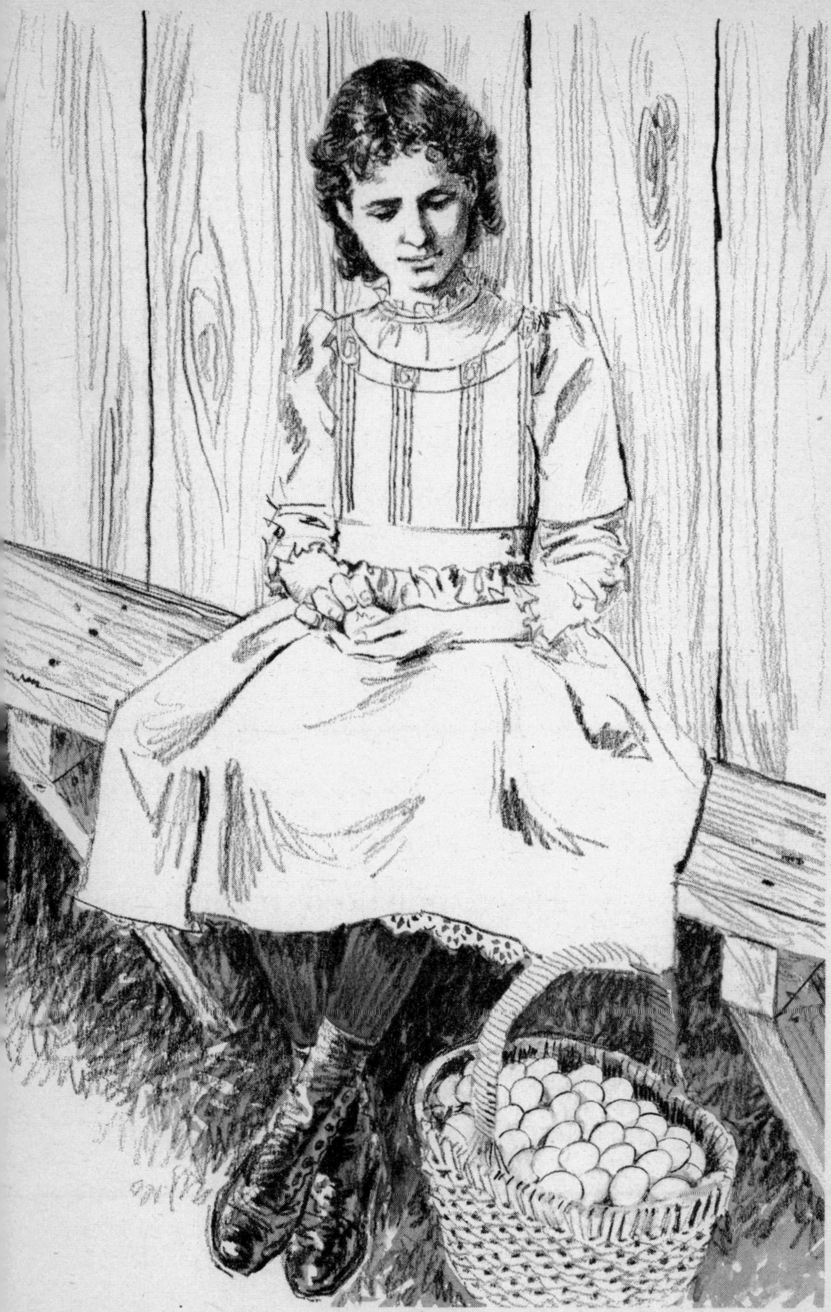

cards. On each card Helen could feel some raised dots. She was puzzled. Her fingers touched the dots carefully. Then Annie spelled the letter "A" with her fingers and put Helen's finger on a card. The raised dots on the card meant "A" also. Helen soon began to understand. The dots were another way of spelling words.

This way of reading is called braille. It had been invented by a blind man named Louis Braille. The letters were printed in raised dots so blind people could read with their fingers.

For days Helen practiced reading the braille letters. When she knew them all she put three cards together and spelled "D-O-G." She ran to find Belle and made the dog's paws touch the letters.

One morning Helen spelled a whole sentence to surprise Annie. "D-O-L-L I-S O-N B-E-D." Annie promised, "Tomorrow you shall have your first book in braille and start reading."

Helen had other important things to learn. She learned to dress herself neatly and make her own bed. She picked up her toys. She learned to be gentle with her little sister. She did not hit Belle or squeeze the kittens.

Sometimes Helen's old tempers came back. But when she touched Teacher's face and felt her mouth turn down Helen knew she had been naughty. Helen's worst punishment was when Annie would not spell stories to her. Annie had taught Helen to love books as much as she did.

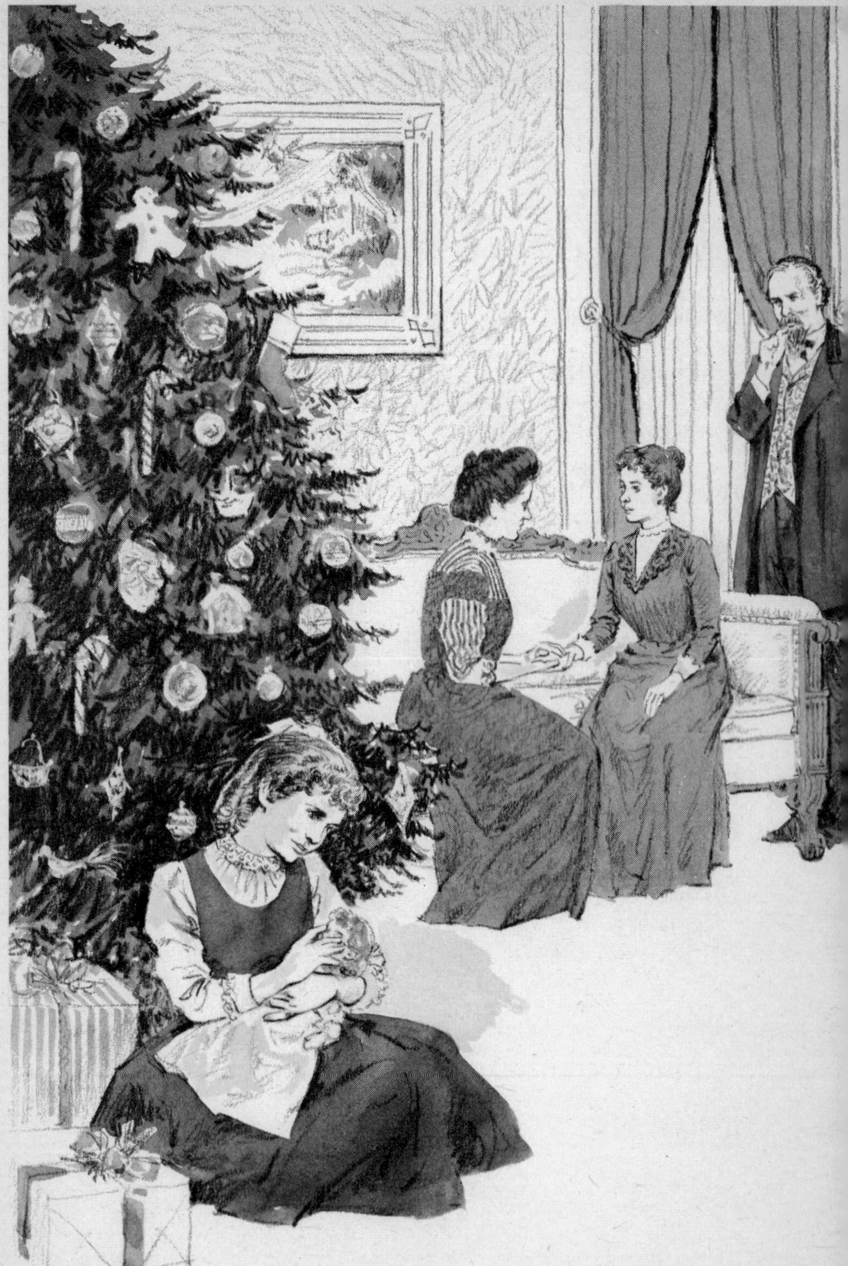

When Christmas came Helen helped make spicy cookies. It was the first Christmas she had understood. She smelled the tree and helped trim its pine branches. Annie helped her wrap presents to surprise the family.

On Christmas night Captain and Mrs. Keller looked at Helen. She sat under the tree holding her new doll. Her face was full of love and joy and understanding.

Mrs. Keller took Annie's hand. "Miss Annie," she said, "I thank God every day of my life for sending you to us."

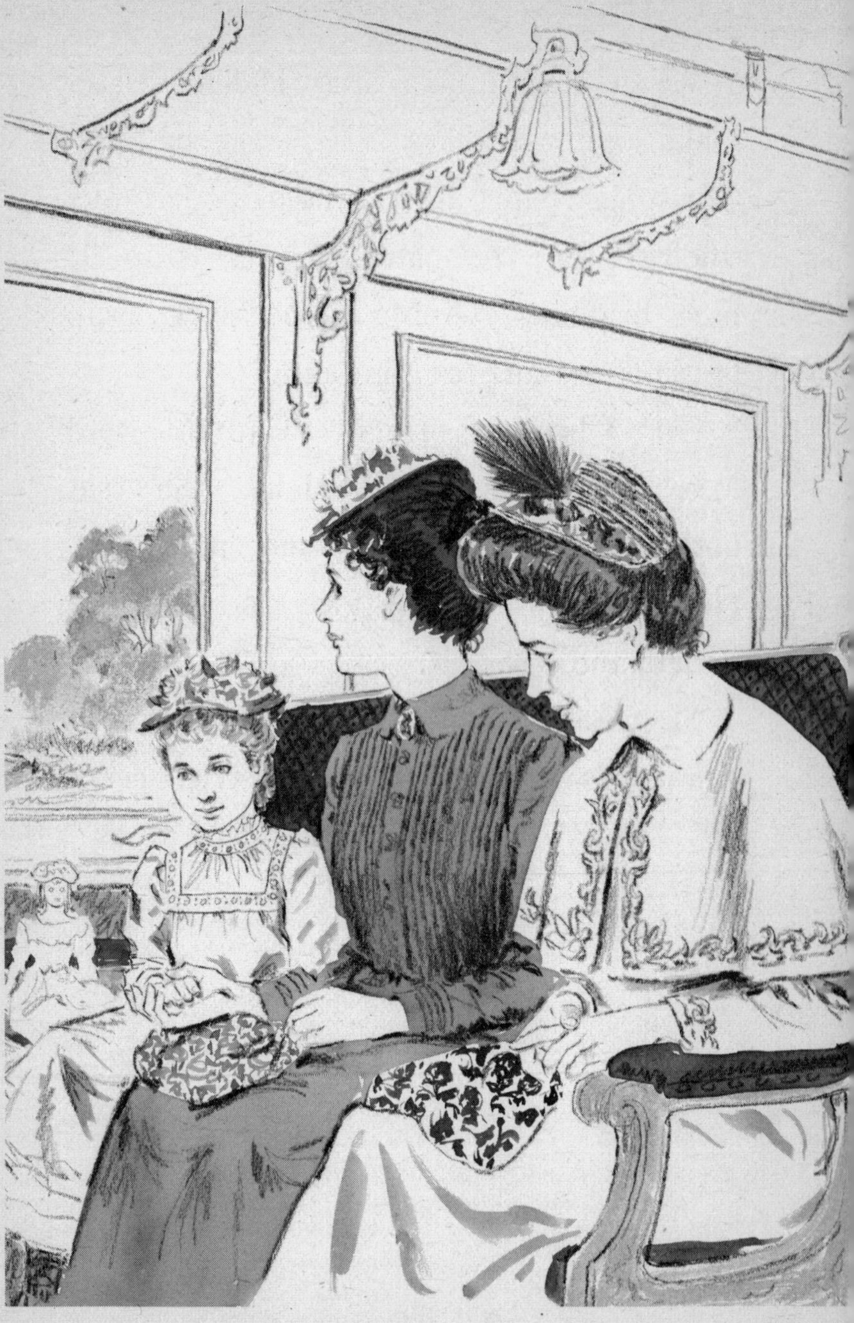

Chapter 5

"I Can Speak!"

Just before Helen's eighth birthday her mother and Teacher took her to Massachusetts. They visited Boston and the seashore at Cape Cod.

It was very different from Helen's last trip by train. Now she understood where they were going. She sat by the window and spelled questions about everything they passed. Annie spelled the answers into Helen's hand. Often she spelled out a joke and they both laughed. They could spell back and forth almost as fast as other people could talk with their voices.

Helen had brought her favorite doll, Nancy, and some of her braille books. When her mother and Annie wanted to rest, Helen curled up with Nancy and read a story to herself. Once a friend asked Helen why she loved books so much.

"Because they tell me about things I cannot see," Helen answered. "And they are never tired or troubled like people."

At the seashore Helen could not wait to run to the beach. The sand was warm on her feet. She felt the roar and crash of the sea and jumped with excitement. Before Annie could stop her she ran straight into a big wave. She tumbled head over heels and came out spluttering.

"Who put salt in the water?" Helen spelled. Her mother and Annie laughed. Soon Helen could jump through waves safely.

When summer ended Mrs. Keller went home. Helen and Annie stayed in Boston. Dr. Anagnos had asked Helen to be a pupil at the Perkins Institute. Annie was still Helen's special teacher. But Helen had some lessons in class-rooms. She made friends quickly with the blind children.

It was the first time Helen had friends her own age. They could spell to her and understand her fingers.

Helen played dolls with the girls. She learned outdoor games. "London Bridge" and tag were her favorites. Helen loved to run fast.

There began to be stories in the newspapers about the little girl from Alabama. People were amazed that a deaf and blind child could read and understand words. Many teachers and important people came to visit Helen. Even Queen Victoria, across the sea in England, heard of her.

Annie was worried. "Helen is becoming a very famous little girl," she told Dr. Anagnos. "I am afraid that so much attention will spoil her."

Helen was too busy to know that anyone was worried. She was studying Latin and German and arithmetic. She

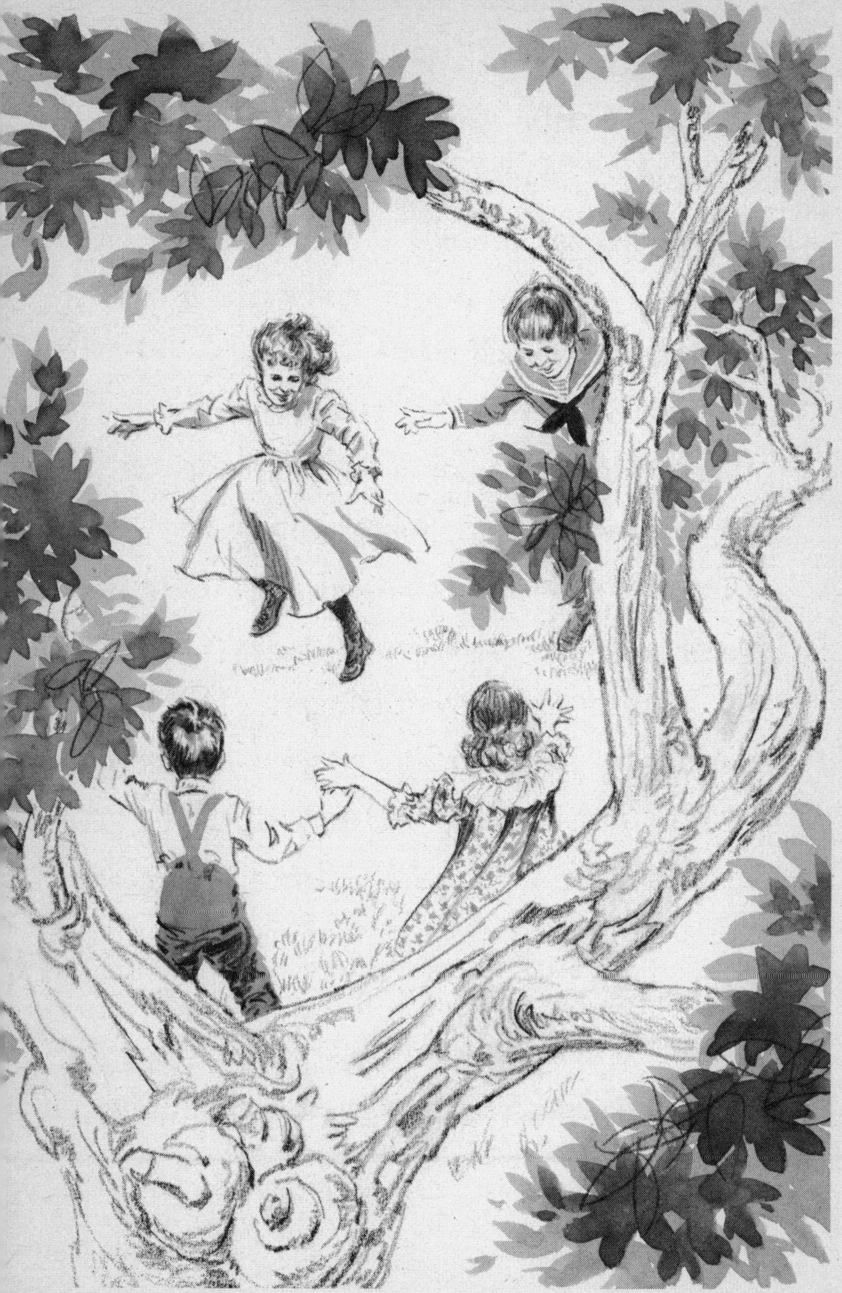

discovered dozens of stories she could read in braille in the school library.

"Helen gobbles books like cookies," Dr. Anagnos smiled. "She cannot get enough." Helen began to write stories and poems herself.

When winter came Helen helped the other children make a snow man. She loved coasting and tobogganing.

In Helen's second year at Perkins school she heard of a little blind-deaf boy named Tommy Stringer. He had no family and no one to teach him.

"We must help," Helen spelled to Annie. They gave a party to raise money to help bring Tommy to the Perkins school. Helen was his special friend. When Tommy learned to spell his first words, Helen was proud of him.

When Helen was ten years old she had a new hope. She heard that a blind-deaf girl in Norway had been taught to use her own voice and speak clearly. Helen wanted to learn to speak herself.

Miss Sarah Fuller gave Helen lessons. She was a teacher at the Horace Mann School for the Deaf in Boston. First Helen would put her hand on Miss Fuller's face when she talked. Then Helen would try to copy the way Miss Fuller's lips and tongue moved.

It was hard work. Over and over Helen tried to make the sounds of M, P, S, A, T and the other letters. But she could not hear the sounds she made. She did not know when her voice sounded queer to others.

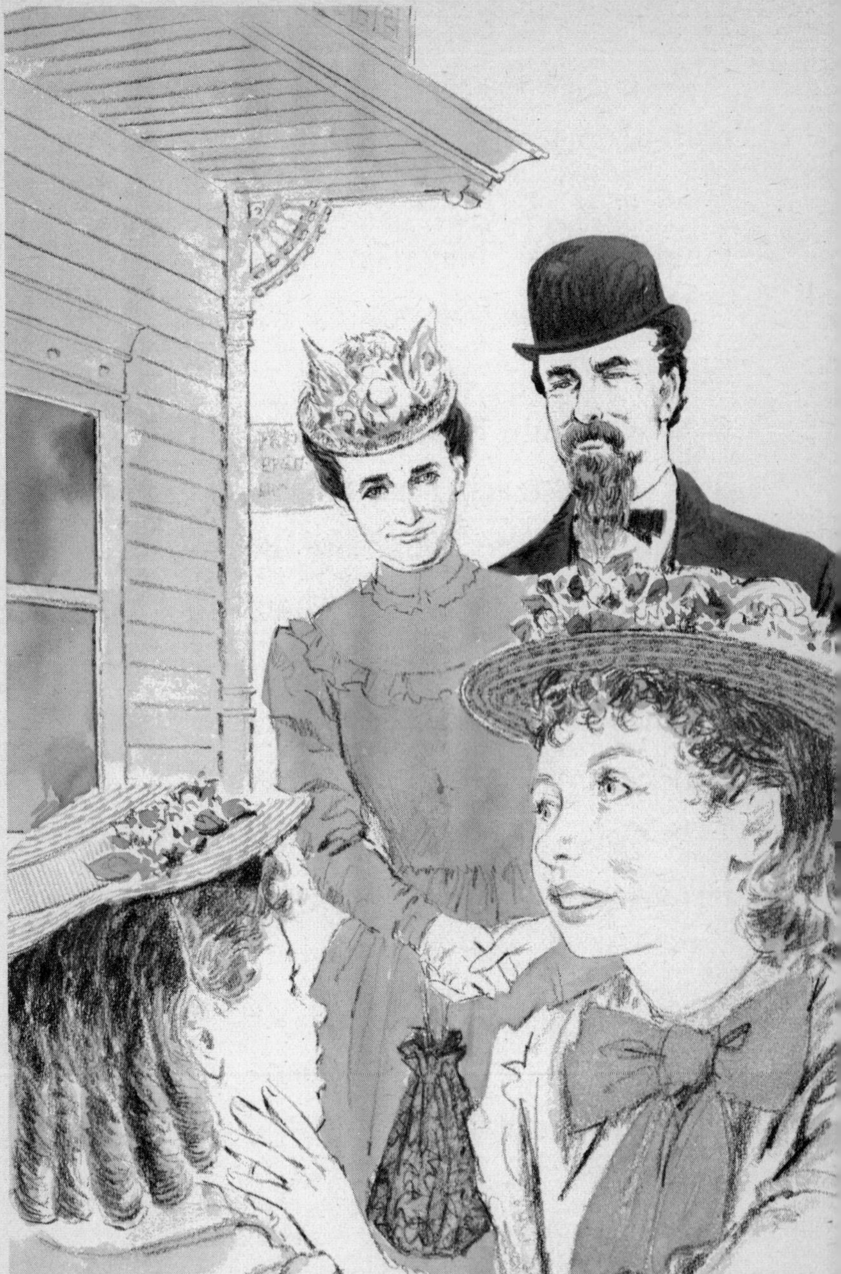

After each lesson, Helen practiced with Annie. At last, one day, she could speak a whole sentence that Annie could understand. They were both overjoyed.

Helen was going home for vacation. She could not wait to show her family that she could truly speak. On the train to Alabama she practiced saying, "Hello, Father and Mother. Hello, Mildred."

The family met Helen and Annie at the station. When they heard Helen speak they hugged her with love and pride.

Driving home, Helen planned one more surprise. At the front steps she jumped out of the carriage first.

"Come, Belle—" she called. When the old dog trotted up and licked her hand, Helen cried happily, "Now Belle can understand me too!"

Chapter 6

College

The year Helen was fourteen she went to the Wright-Humason School in New York. Annie sat beside Helen in classes. She spelled the teacher's words into Helen's hand.

Dr. Humason gave Helen special lessons in speaking and lip reading. She learned to put her fingers on other people's lips and understand what they were saying.

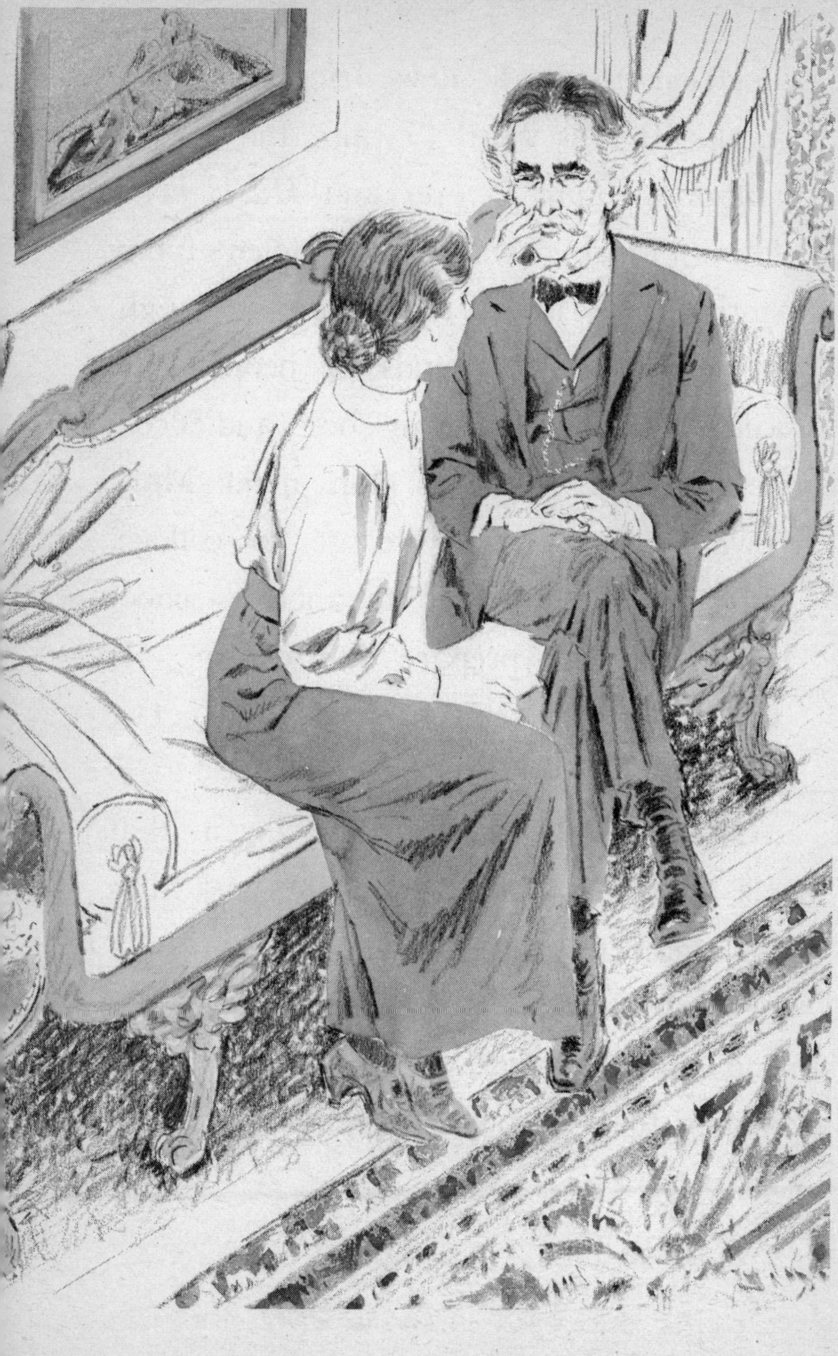

Helen made a new friend in New York. It was Mark Twain, the famous author of *Tom Sawyer* and *Huckleberry Finn*. Mark Twain told Helen funny stories. He loved to make her laugh. "I lecture to thousands of people," he said, "but Helen is my best audience."

Helen had a serious plan to tell Mark Twain. She wanted to go to college. But first she must go to another school and study to prepare for college. It would mean long, hard work. The school would be expensive.

Helen explained to Mark Twain that her father was ill. "I cannot ask him for the extra money," she said.

Mark Twain encouraged Helen. He and some of her other friends raised money to help pay her school expenses.

"I will work hard," Helen promised. She studied at the Gilman School in Boston and with private teachers. She used a braille typewriter to keep her study notes. She learned to use a regular typewriter for her school papers.

Shortly before examination time, sad news came from Helen's home. Her father, Captain Keller, had died. It was hard for Helen to go on studying. She longed to go home and comfort her mother and sister.

Annie was not allowed to go into the examination room with Helen. A teacher spelled the questions into Helen's hand. Then Helen typed the answers.

The next week Helen heard that she had passed all her subjects. She would enter Radcliffe College in the fall of

1900. She could join her family and rest for the summer.

When college classes began Annie sat next to Helen. She spelled what the teachers said into Helen's hand. Annie looked up words in the dictionary for Helen. She read Helen books that were not printed in braille.

The girls in Helen's class were friendly. They elected her vice-president of the class.

English was Helen's favorite subject. She wrote such good themes that some were published in a book. A magazine paid her to write the story of her life. Helen was glad she could earn money.

A young teacher named John Macy helped Helen with her writing. He was soon a friend of both Helen and Annie.

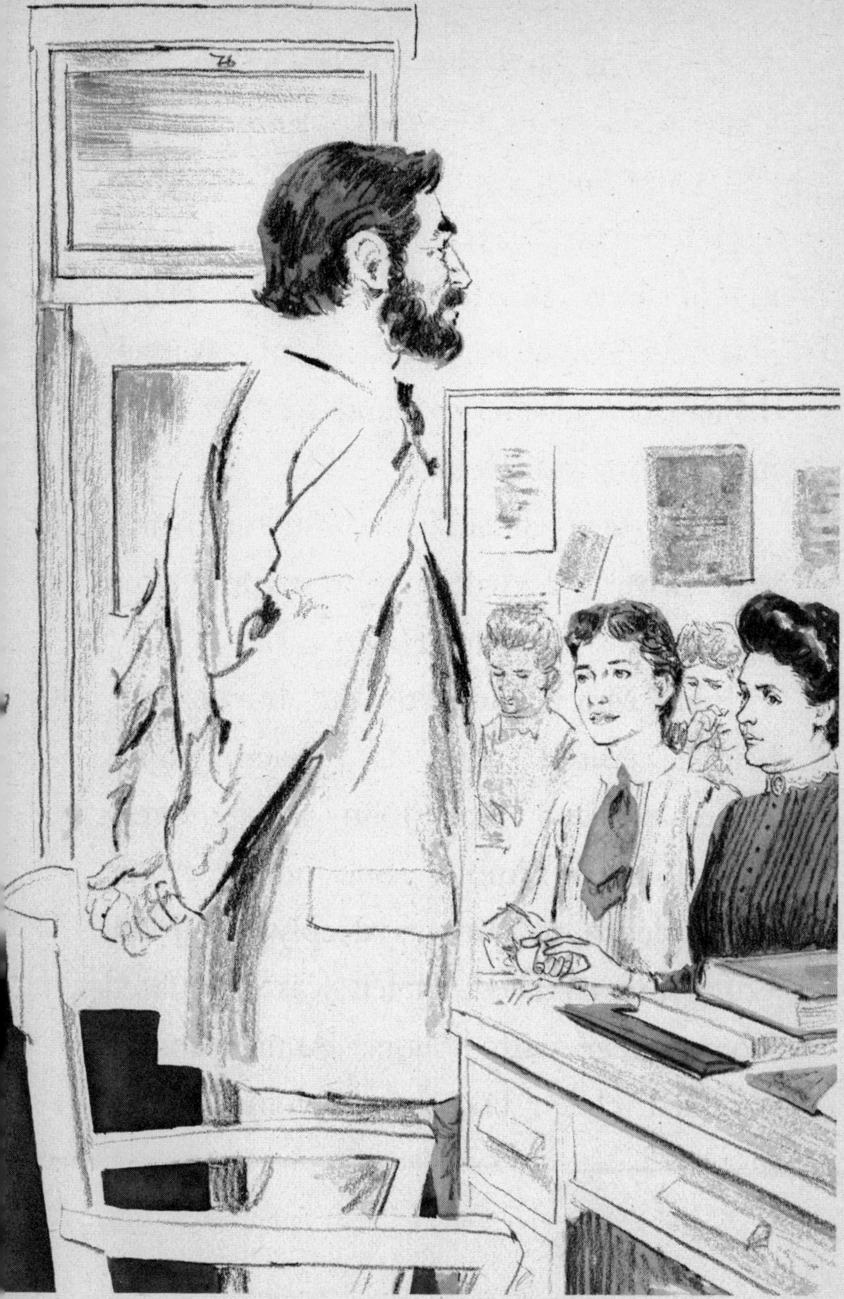

They went boating together on the Charles River. They took picnic lunches and went hiking in the woods.

Helen's last year of college work was the hardest. Beside her studying, Helen now had Annie to worry about. Annie's delicate eyes were red and sore from all her reading to Helen.

Helen begged Annie to rest, but Annie was firm. "I will not rest until you graduate," she told Helen.

John Macy came to the rescue. He helped Annie read to Helen. Soon Helen realized that John was growing very fond of Annie. She hoped Annie would learn to care as deeply for John.

In June of 1904, Helen was graduated from college with honors. Annie proudly watched Helen take her diploma.

Chapter 7

A New Career

Helen and Annie went to live in Wrentham, near Boston. John Macy still came to see them often.

On one bright May afternoon Helen stood beside Teacher as Anne Sullivan and John Macy were married.

Helen was very happy about the marriage. Annie and John lived in Wrentham with her. Now the three planned to work together.

Helen had a hard time deciding what work would be best for her. "You should teach," many of her friends advised her.

Helen wanted to pass on the gift of teaching that Annie had given her. But at last she decided she could work best by writing and lecturing. "I can tell more people about the special training that deaf and blind children need," she told Annie. "I can teach them what you taught me—that children must not be different because they are blind or deaf. They can learn to work and be happy."

Before she began to lecture, Helen took more voice lessons. She practiced for many hours so that people could understand her speeches.

During the next years Helen and Annie lectured to big audiences all over the country. Traveling on trains and meeting thousands of strangers was hard work. But they were happy when they saw new schools being started and new organizations helping to educate the blind and deaf.

Between trips Helen wrote books and articles for magazines. After each long trip she was happy to come home to Wrentham. She always went first to the garden and put her arms around her favorite trees. Her Great Dane dog and the puppies barked their welcome.

Helen and Annie rode horseback over the country trails. She and Annie and John spent long evenings by the fire with their friends.

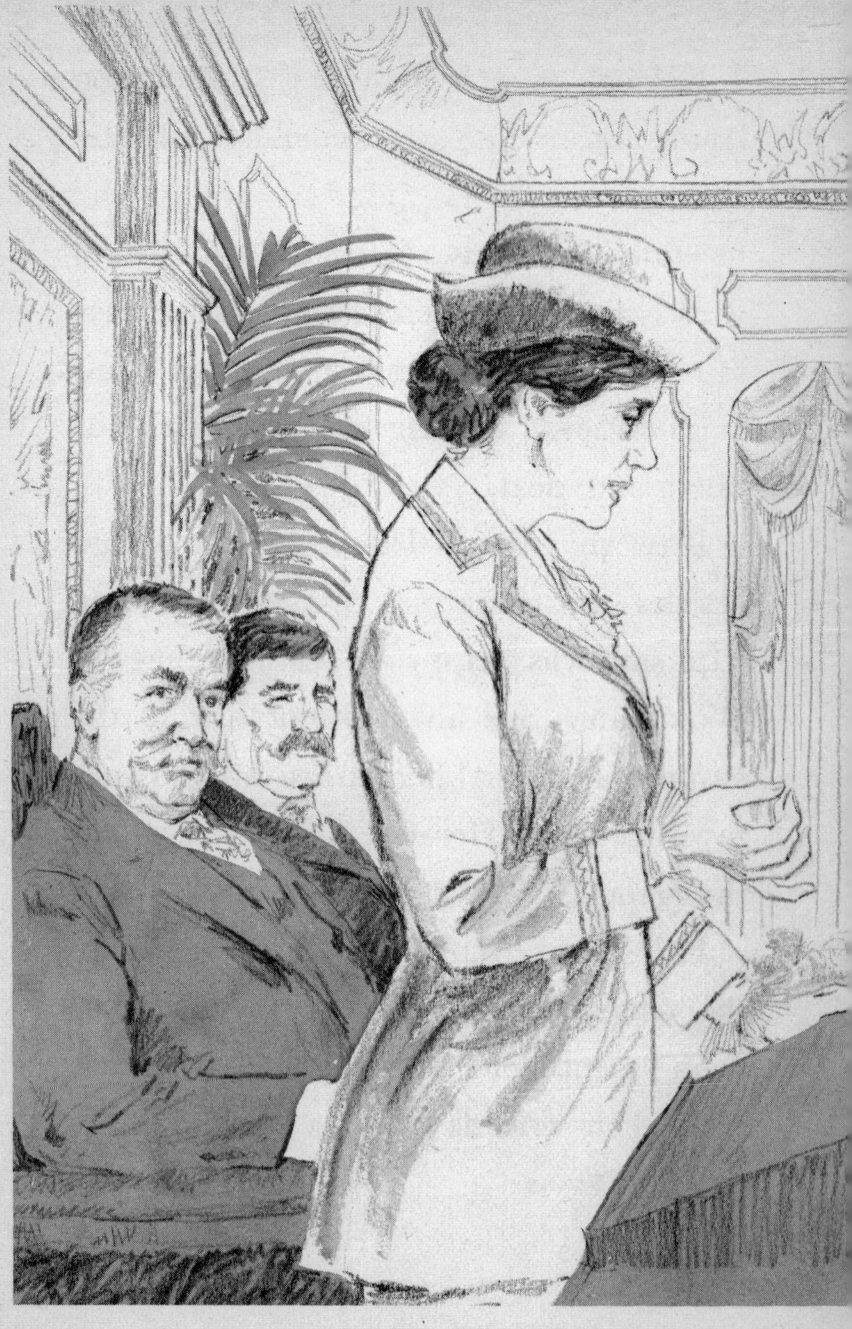

Helen had always worked to get more books printed in braille. She knew that many blind people did not have enough books to read. She went to Washington to ask people in the government to help.

In 1913 there was important news. The National Library for the Blind was started. Helen and Annie went to Washington again. President Taft of the United States opened the new library.

Later Helen met President Taft again. He came to New York to open the first Lighthouse for the Blind. Helen made a speech. She welcomed the new group that would work for the blind.

That night, when they had supper by the fire, Helen smiled.

"We started long ago with little Tommy Stringer," she told Annie. "We have traveled until our bones ached. We have talked ourselves hoarse to tell people that blind and deaf children need special schools. People have *listened*. Now some of our dreams are coming true."

A few years later trouble came. Annie was ill. Her marriage with John Macy had become unhappy. When John left Wrentham Annie and Helen missed him sadly.

At the same time Helen's work grew so heavy that she and Annie needed more help. A young Scottish girl named Polly Thompson came to live with them. Polly was quick and sensible and jolly. She could cook and give the dogs baths. She helped Helen with writing and reading to rest Annie's eyes.

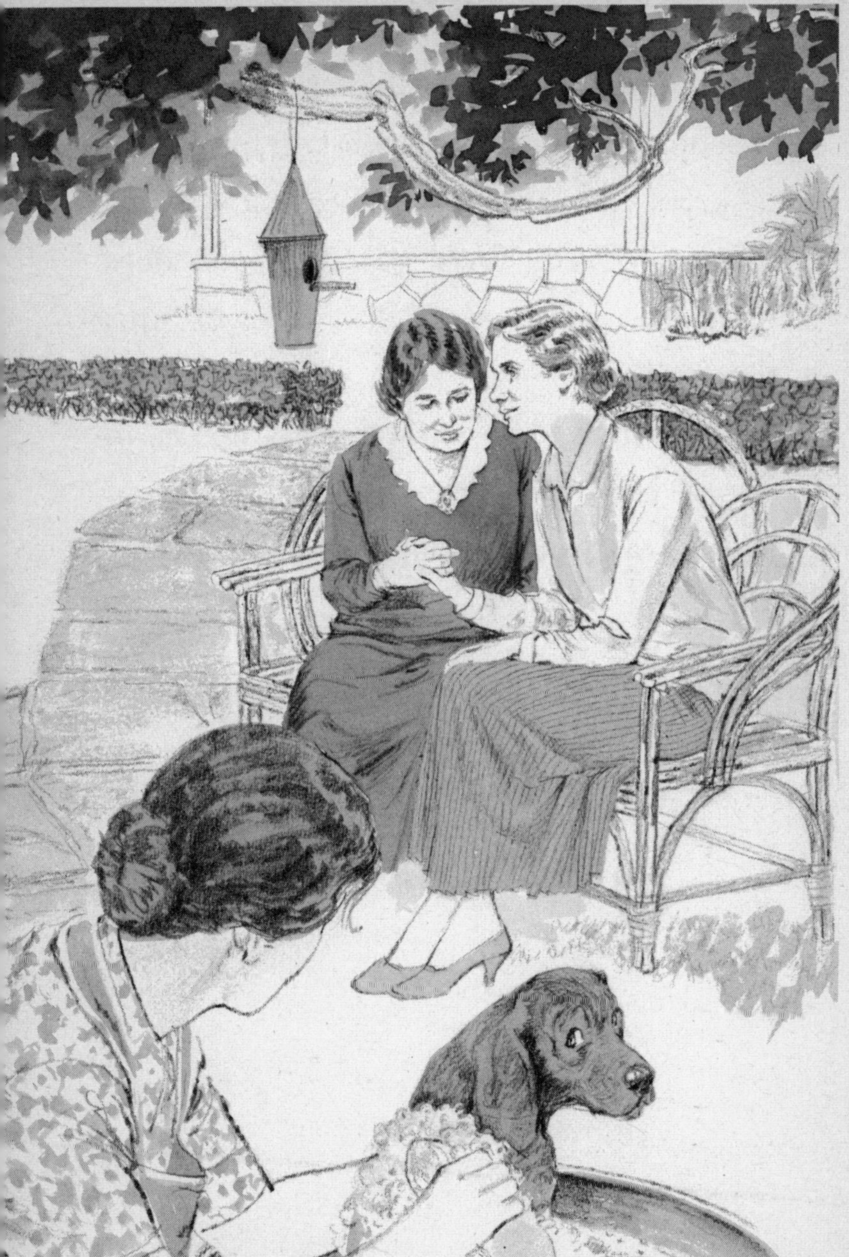

Without John's help, the house in Wrentham was too expensive for Helen to keep. She was sad to leave the home she had loved. "We can take the dogs with us," she said. "But we will miss the garden."

They moved to a smaller house in Forest Hills, near New York City. Soon Helen was working hard on a new book.

Chapter 8

War

In 1917 the United States entered World War I in Europe. The roar of faraway guns brought more changes to Helen Keller's life.

Helen had to give up many of her lecture trips. She and Teacher were very unhappy over the sad war news. They grieved for the many soldiers who were killed or wounded.

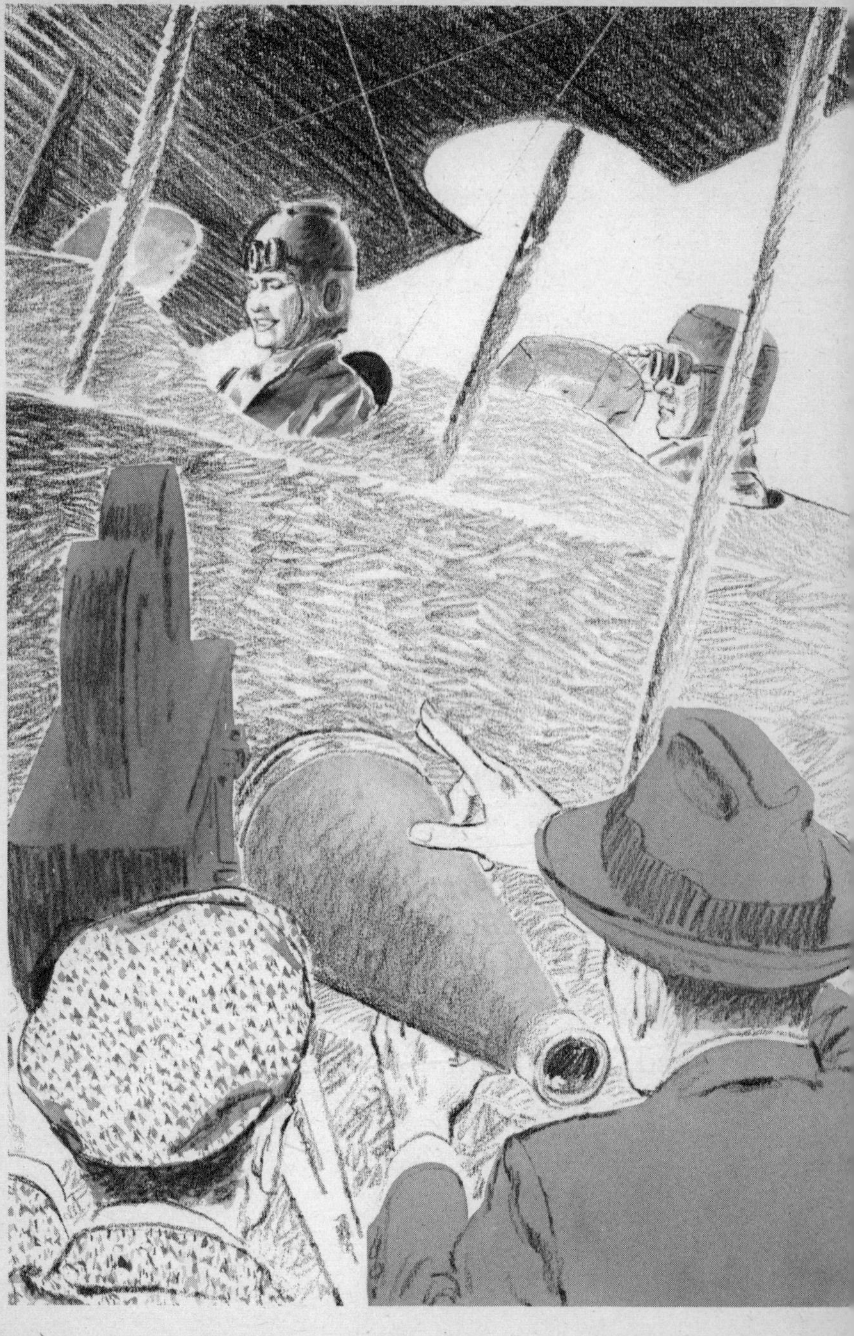

Shortly after the war ended, Helen was asked to act in a movie. It would tell the story of her life.

"A new adventure will be good for us," Helen said. She still needed more money to take care of herself and Annie and Polly. They traveled to California.

The movie work was exciting. In one scene Helen had to fly in an open plane. It did daring stunts. In another scene she rode a frisky horse that nearly threw her off.

Annie and Polly gave Helen a new nickname. They called her "Daredevil Helen."

Soon afterward Helen and Annie were asked to do an act together on the stage. They were to appear in theaters all over the country.

They were both nervous the first time the curtain rolled up. The spotlights were bright. Annie came on the stage first and told about Helen's early life. When Helen came on the audience always clapped.

Helen read Annie's lips and answered questions from the audience. Some of them were foolish.

"Do you shut your eyes when you go to sleep?"

"I never stayed awake to find out," Helen answered.

The act was a success. Helen and Annie earned the money they needed.

Now Helen could work again for others. She was happy with news from Washington. Congress had voted money for many more books for the blind.

Some could be played on records. They were called "talking books."

The American Foundation for the Blind was an active new group. Helen went to work for the Foundation.

Helen Keller was famous around the world now. She had met people from every country. She had been invited to visit every President in the White House since her childhood.

But darkness was closing in again. Helen's mother had died, and Annie became very ill. The year was 1936. Annie was 70 years old. Her eyes were worn out with work. She was almost blind. But she had seen Helen succeed. She had seen new work for the blind beginning all over the country, much of it from Helen and Annie's work.

Annie was sick for many months. Long nights Helen sat beside her. She and Polly nursed Annie tenderly.

Helen held Teacher's hand when she died. Helen felt as if her own life had ended. They had been together almost 50 years.

It was the saddest time of Helen's life. "A light has gone out that can never shine for me again," she said.

Chapter 9

Around the World

Many people wrote Helen letters of sympathy. One from a stranger began: *"I know, dear Helen Keller, your heart is crying out for the loved one. Our only comfort is to do what good we can in this world."*

Helen was deeply touched. She felt as if Annie's own words were reaching her through the stranger's letter. "We must stop feeling sad and get back to work," she told Polly.

Soon afterward an important telegram came. The Japanese government asked Helen to help start work for their blind and deaf. This meant a long trip across the Pacific Ocean. Helen knew she must give many speeches.

"I cannot say no," Helen said. "There are many thousands of deaf and blind children in Japan. Most of them have no teachers. We must help raise money to start schools for them, just as we are doing in America."

On the ship, crossing the ocean, Helen wrote the speeches she would give in Japan. She and Polly got up at five o'clock each morning to go out on deck alone. Then Helen would practice her speeches so Polly could tell her if her voice sounded right.

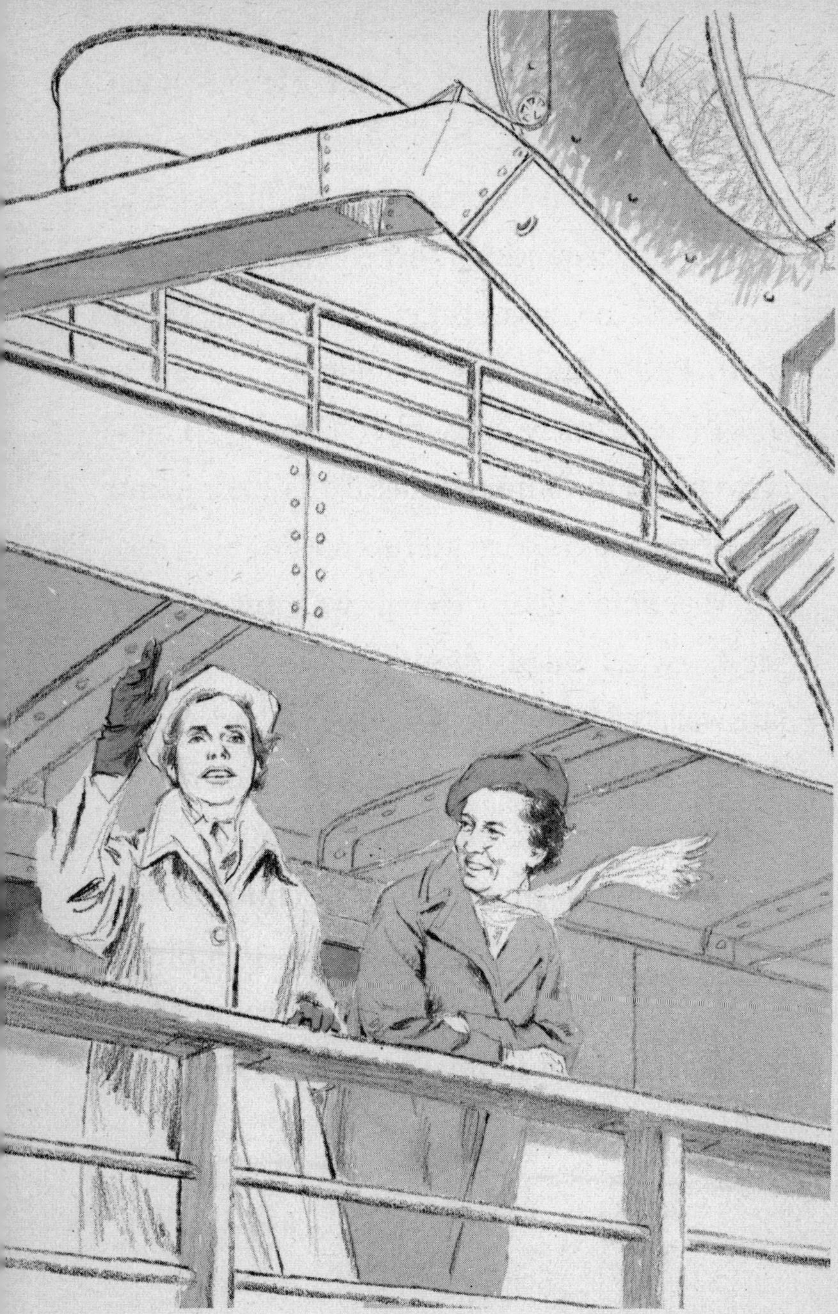

In Japan crowds greeted Helen. They threw flowers in front of her car. Best of all, Helen liked the children who gathered around to greet her.

When it was time to leave, Helen and Polly had raised enough money to begin the new schools. The Japanese government thanked them. The Emperor of Japan sent a grateful message.

At home again Helen was busy. Her desk was piled high with letters to answer. Many parents who had blind or deaf children wrote to Helen for advice. She answered them all.

Helen was proud of the children she had helped. Tommy Stringer, the blind-deaf boy, was now a tall, strong man. He earned his living as a carpenter. He had a family of his own.

One day a friend of Helen's came home from a walk. "I did not see anything interesting," she said. Helen was amazed. It made her think how much she wished she could see—even for a little while. Later she wrote a magazine article called *"If I Had Three Days To See."*

Helen wrote that first she would want to see the faces of her family and friends she loved. Then she wanted to see her house and her books and her dogs. She would go for a long walk through the woods. She wished that she could see a sunset, and children playing, and the moon and stars. She wanted to see a stage play and a funny movie.

While Helen worked she thought of Teacher's empty room next to her study.

It made her feel lonely again. Soon she and Polly moved to a new house in Westport, Connecticut.

The shadow of war was over the country again. Fighting had begun in Europe. America entered the war in 1941. Helen and Polly were sad that Japan was now America's enemy. They remembered their Japanese friends.

Many soldiers and sailors were blinded in the fighting. President Roosevelt asked Helen to visit them. She traveled to hospitals all over the country.

"You can learn to read and to work again," she told the men. "You must learn to be a part of the world and not outside of it." Her words and her gentle touch brought them new courage and hope.

Chapter 10

Peace

In 1945 the long war ended. The next year Helen and Polly went to Europe to help the blind there.

One evening in Rome Helen felt the quick excitement of Polly's hand. Polly was spelling terrible news. Their house in Westport had been burned. Everything was lost.

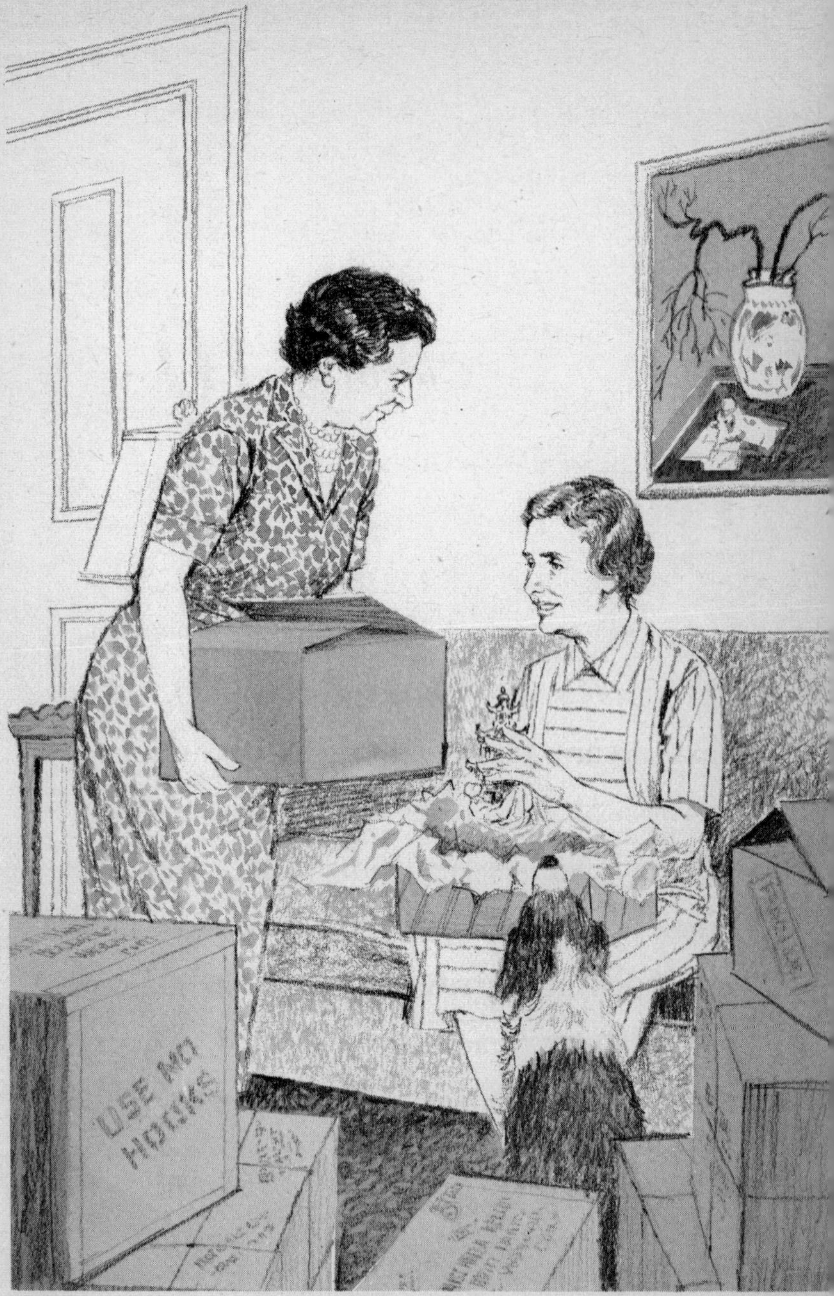
USE NO HOOKS

Worst of all, a book Helen had been writing about Teacher had burned. It had been nearly finished. "The very first thing I will do is start the book over again," Helen said.

Back in Westport, Helen's loyal friends helped build a new house. The day Helen and Polly moved into their new home, huge boxes arrived. Helen's friends in Japan had heard of her loss. They had sent gifts of tables and lamps and other furniture.

Helen ran her fingers over the delicate china and carvings. One package was wrapped the most beautifully. It was a tall incense burner. The Emperor had sent it to his friend, Helen Keller.

Many honors came to Helen Keller through the years. Colleges all over the world gave her special honors. Many foreign governments gave her medals and decorations.

Most important, Helen saw more and more blind and deaf people educated to do useful work and be a part of the living world. Much of the help had come from her. Great countries, and little children, gave Helen their thanks.

In May, 1959, Helen was given the honor she prized most. The Helen Keller World Crusade was begun at the United Nations building in New York City. It would help blind and deaf children all over the world.

Helen was very proud. She had lived through two terrible world wars. She had always hoped for world peace. Now it made her happy to know that people of different countries and races would work together to help children.

Long after the time when most people retire, Helen Keller was busy. "I cannot stop to grow old while there is so much work to do," she said, "and so many children to help."

When Helen was 75 she traveled thousands of miles around the world. She made many speeches and met many new friends.

On her eightieth birthday, in 1960, the American Foundation for Overseas Blind announced the Helen Keller International Award. This was for people who had given outstanding help to the blind. There is also a Helen Keller Scholarship for deaf-blind students to help them go to college.

Now Helen Keller could no longer travel herself. But her spirit of courage and the words of her books still travel around the world.

Helen never forgot that all of her work and all of her honors and all the light in her life came first from her beloved Teacher. One of Helen Keller's most beautiful books is the story of Anne Sullivan Macy's life. In a little verse Helen wrote:

"Teacher—and that was all.
It will be my answer
In the dark
When death calls."